CHAPTER 1
Understanding Diabetes

Diabetes is a complex metabolic disorder characterised by elevated blood sugar levels, affecting millions of individuals worldwide. Understanding the intricacies of diabetes is crucial for effective management and prevention.

1. Diabetes Defined:

- Definition of Diabetes Mellitus
- Insulin and its Role
- Hyperglycemia: The Core Challenge

2. Types of Diabetes:

- Type 1 Diabetes:
    - Causes and Onset
    - Autoimmune Component
    - Insulin Dependency
- Type 2 Diabetes:
    - Insulin Resistance
    - Lifestyle Factors
    - Genetic Predisposition
- Gestational Diabetes:
    - Occurrence during Pregnancy
    - Risk Factors
    - Implications for Mother and Child
- Other Types and Variants:
    - LADA (Latent Autoimmune Diabetes in Adults)
    - MODY (Maturity-Onset Diabetes of the Young)
    - Secondary Diabetes

Diabetes mellitus is a chronic metabolic disorder characterised by elevated blood glucose levels, resulting from either insufficient insulin production, impaired insulin utilisation, or a combination of both. This condition profoundly impacts the body's ability to regulate blood sugar, leading to various complications if left unmanaged.

Key Components:

Insulin and Glucose:
- Insulin, produced by the pancreas, plays a vital role in regulating blood sugar.
- Glucose, derived from the food we consume, serves as the primary source of energy for the body.

Hyperglycemia:
- Diabetes is marked by persistent hyperglycemia, an elevated level of glucose in the blood.
- The inability to effectively move glucose into cells leads to an accumulation in the bloodstream.

Types of Diabetes Mellitus:

- Type 1 Diabetes:
  - Autoimmune destruction of insulin-producing beta cells.
  - Typically diagnosed in childhood or adolescence.
  - Requires lifelong insulin therapy.
- Type 2 Diabetes:
  - Insulin resistance and impaired insulin secretion.
  - Commonly develops in adulthood, but can occur at any age.
  - Managed through lifestyle changes, medications, and insulin in some cases.
- Gestational Diabetes:
  - Occurs during pregnancy, affecting blood sugar levels.
  - Increases the risk of developing type 2 diabetes later in life.

Latent Autoimmune Diabetes in Adults, commonly known as LADA, represents a unique form of diabetes that shares characteristics of both type 1 and type 2 diabetes. LADA is characterised by a slower onset of autoimmune destruction of insulin-producing beta cells, typically affecting adults.

Key Features:

Autoimmune Component:
- Similar to type 1 diabetes, LADA involves an autoimmune response where the body's immune system attacks and gradually destroys insulin-producing beta cells in the pancreas.

Age of Onset:
- LADA typically emerges in adulthood, distinguishing it from the more common age of onset for type 1 diabetes, which often occurs in childhood or adolescence.

Insulin Dependency:
- While LADA initially presents with features of type 2 diabetes, individuals with LADA often become insulin-dependent over time as the autoimmune destruction progresses.

Clinical Presentation:
- LADA may initially be misdiagnosed as type 2 diabetes due to its gradual onset and presentation in adults. However, closer monitoring may reveal a decline in insulin production.

Diagnosis and Management:

Autoantibody Testing:
- Diagnosis often involves testing for autoantibodies associated with autoimmune diabetes, such as GAD antibodies (glutamic acid decarboxylase).

Treatment Approach:

- LADA management may start with oral medications commonly used for type 2 diabetes. However, insulin therapy becomes necessary as beta cell function declines.

Prognosis and Considerations:

Progression:
- LADA progression varies among individuals. Some may maintain partial beta cell function for an extended period, while others may require insulin relatively soon after diagnosis.

Risk Factors:
- Individuals with LADA may have a genetic predisposition to autoimmune diabetes, and certain environmental factors could contribute to its development.

Maturity-Onset Diabetes of the Young, abbreviated as MODY, is a rare and inherited form of diabetes characterised by a monogenic (single gene) mutation affecting insulin production. Unlike more common types of diabetes, MODY typically manifests at a younger age and often runs in families.

Key Features:

Genetic Basis:
- MODY results from a mutation in a single gene, disrupting the normal function of beta cells in the pancreas, which are responsible for insulin production.

Early Onset:
- Unlike type 1 and type 2 diabetes, MODY usually presents at a younger age, often during adolescence or early adulthood.

Familial Inheritance:
- MODY is often inherited in an autosomal dominant pattern, meaning that a child has a 50% chance of inheriting the mutated gene from a parent with MODY.

Insulin Production Affected:

- The genetic mutations in MODY primarily impact the ability of beta cells to produce insulin. This distinguishes it from other types of diabetes with more complex and multifactorial causes.

Types of MODY:

MODY Subtypes:
- There are several subtypes of MODY, each associated with specific genes. Common subtypes include MODY 2 (glucokinase gene mutation) and MODY 3 (HNF1A gene mutation).

Diagnosis and Management:

Genetic Testing:
- Diagnosis of MODY involves genetic testing to identify the specific mutation causing the condition.

Tailored Treatment:
- Treatment for MODY is often more specific, taking into account the underlying genetic cause. Medications and insulin therapy may be prescribed based on the subtype and individual needs.

Prognosis and Considerations:

Stable Blood Sugar Levels:
- MODY individuals may have more stable blood sugar levels compared to other forms of diabetes.

Risk for Family Members:
- Family members of an individual with MODY may undergo genetic testing to determine their risk of carrying the mutated gene.

Prevalence and Global Impact of Diabetes:

Introduction:

Understanding the prevalence and global impact of diabetes is crucial in addressing the scale of this chronic health condition that affects individuals, families, and healthcare systems worldwide.

1. Epidemiological Landscape:

- Overview of the increasing prevalence of diabetes globally.
- Statistics on the number of people affected by diabetes across different age groups.

2. Regional Variances:

- Examination of regional differences in diabetes prevalence.
- Factors contributing to variations, including genetic predisposition, lifestyle, and healthcare access.

3. Societal and Economic Impact:

- Discussion on the broader implications of diabetes on societies and economies.
- Impact on healthcare costs, productivity, and quality of life for individuals and communities.

4. Rise of Type 2 Diabetes:

- Exploration of the significant increase in type 2 diabetes cases.
- Link between lifestyle factors, urbanisation, and the surge in type 2 diabetes prevalence.

5. Global Health Disparities:

- Analysis of disparities in diabetes prevalence based on socio-economic factors.
- Access to healthcare, education, and cultural influences contributing to health inequalities.

6. Complications and Healthcare Burden:

- Overview of the health complications associated with diabetes.
- Analysis of the burden on healthcare systems, including hospitalisation rates and healthcare expenditure.

7. Impact on Quality of Life:

- Examination of how diabetes affects the daily lives of individuals and their families.
- Emotional, psychological, and social aspects of living with diabetes.

8. Public Health Strategies:

- Discussion on global efforts and initiatives to address the diabetes epidemic.
- Implementation of prevention programs, early detection, and management strategies.

9. Future Projections:

- Examination of projections for diabetes prevalence in the coming years.
- Potential factors influencing future trends and implications for public health planning.

Basics of Diabetes:

Introduction:

To comprehend diabetes, one must delve into the fundamental aspects that define this complex metabolic disorder, involving the intricate interplay of insulin, glucose, and the body's regulatory mechanisms.

1. Anatomy and Physiology of the Pancreas:

- Overview of the pancreas as a vital organ in diabetes.
- Role of the pancreas in producing insulin and glucagon.

2. Insulin and Glucose:

- In-depth exploration of insulin as a key hormone in blood sugar regulation.
- Understanding glucose as the primary source of energy for the body.

3. How the Body Normally Regulates Blood Sugar:

- Examination of the physiological mechanisms that maintain blood sugar within a narrow range.
- Role of insulin in facilitating glucose uptake by cells.

4. Disruption in Diabetes:

- Explanation of how diabetes arises due to impaired insulin function or insufficient insulin production.
- Disturbance in glucose metabolism leading to hyperglycemia.

5. Risk Factors:

- Identification of risk factors contributing to the development of diabetes.
- Genetic predisposition, lifestyle factors, and other contributors.

6. Symptoms of Diabetes:

- Recognition of common signs indicating the presence of diabetes.

- Polyuria, polydipsia, unexplained weight loss, and other symptoms.

7. Diagnosis:

- Overview of diagnostic tests used to identify diabetes.
- Blood sugar tests, A1C test, and oral glucose tolerance test.

8. Importance of Early Detection:

- Discussion on the significance of early diagnosis in managing diabetes.
- Preventing complications through timely intervention.

9. Pre-diabetes:

- Definition and significance of pre-diabetes as an intermediate stage.
- Lifestyle modifications and prevention strategies.

10. Role of Lifestyle:

- The impact of diet, exercise, and healthy habits in diabetes prevention and management.
- Personalised lifestyle adjustments for optimal blood sugar control.

How the Body Normally Regulates Blood Sugar:

Introduction:

The regulation of blood sugar (glucose) is a finely tuned and dynamic process in the human body, orchestrated by a complex interplay of hormones and organs to maintain a stable internal environment. Here's an overview of how the body typically regulates blood sugar levels:

1. Role of the Pancreas:

- The pancreas, a dual-function organ located behind the stomach, plays a crucial role in blood sugar regulation.
- It contains clusters of cells called the Islets of Langerhans, specifically the beta cells, which produce insulin.

2. Insulin Secretion:

- After a meal, especially one rich in carbohydrates, blood sugar levels rise.
- In response, beta cells release insulin into the bloodstream.

3. Cellular Uptake of Glucose:

- Insulin acts as a key that unlocks cells, allowing glucose to enter.
- Cells utilise glucose for energy, particularly muscle and adipose (fat) cells.

4. Glycogen Storage in the Liver:

- Excess glucose that is not immediately needed for energy is converted into glycogen in the liver.
- The liver acts as a glucose reservoir, releasing stored glucose into the bloodstream when needed.

5. Suppression of Glucose Release:

- Insulin inhibits the liver from releasing too much glucose into the bloodstream.
- This suppression helps prevent excessive elevation of blood sugar levels.

6. Glucagon Counterbalance:

- The pancreas also produces another hormone called glucagon, which has the opposite effect of insulin.
- In between meals or during periods of fasting, glucagon prompts the liver to release stored glucose into the bloodstream.

7. Kidneys and Glucose Reabsorption:

- The kidneys play a role in maintaining blood sugar balance by reabsorbing glucose back into the bloodstream during filtration.
- Under normal circumstances, glucose is not excreted in significant amounts in the urine.

8. Feedback Mechanism:

- Blood sugar levels are continuously monitored by the body.
- If levels deviate from the normal range, the pancreas adjusts insulin and glucagon secretion to bring them back to equilibrium.

9. Cellular Sensitivity to Insulin:

- The responsiveness of cells to insulin is crucial for proper blood sugar regulation.
- In conditions like insulin resistance, cells become less sensitive to insulin, leading to elevated blood sugar levels.

CHAPTER 2

Types of Diabetes

Diabetes is a heterogeneous group of metabolic disorders characterised by elevated blood sugar levels. Understanding the different types of diabetes is crucial for accurate diagnosis and effective management. Here are the primary types:

1. Type 1 Diabetes:

- Cause: Autoimmune destruction of insulin-producing beta cells in the pancreas.
- Onset: Typically diagnosed in childhood or adolescence.
- Treatment: Requires lifelong insulin therapy.

2. Type 2 Diabetes:

- Cause: Combination of insulin resistance and impaired insulin secretion.
- Onset: Commonly develops in adulthood but can occur at any age.
- Treatment: Managed through lifestyle changes, oral medications, and, in some cases, insulin.

3. Gestational Diabetes:

- Occurrence: Develops during pregnancy.
- Cause: Insufficient insulin production to meet increased needs during pregnancy.
- Risk: Increases the risk of type 2 diabetes later in life for both mother and child.
- Management: Dietary changes, monitoring, and sometimes insulin therapy.

4. LADA (Latent Autoimmune Diabetes in Adults):

- Characteristics: Slow onset autoimmune diabetes in adults.
- Similarity to Type 1: Shares autoimmune features with type 1 diabetes.
- Insulin Dependency: Individuals may become insulin-dependent over time.

5. MODY (Maturity-Onset Diabetes of the Young):

- Genetic Basis: Caused by mutations in a single gene.
- Onset: Typically diagnosed in adolescence or early adulthood.
- Inheritance: Often inherited in an autosomal dominant pattern.

6. Secondary Diabetes:

- Cause: Result of another medical condition or factor, such as certain medications, diseases, or pancreatic disorders.
- Management: Addressing the underlying cause is crucial.

7. Type 3 Diabetes (Alzheimer's Disease):

- Link: Proposed association between insulin resistance in the brain and the development of Alzheimer's disease.
- Research: Ongoing research into the connection between diabetes and cognitive decline.

8. Type 1.5 Diabetes:

- Characteristics: Term sometimes used to describe LADA due to its features overlapping with both type 1 and type 2 diabetes.

- Management: Often involves a combination of lifestyle changes and insulin therapy.

Diabetes Management during Pregnancy:

Introduction:

Pregnancy introduces unique considerations for women with diabetes, as it can impact blood sugar levels and pose potential risks for both the mother and the developing baby. Effective management is essential to ensure a healthy pregnancy and minimise complications. Here's an overview of diabetes management during pregnancy:

1. Preconception Planning:

- Optimal Blood Sugar Levels: Achieving and maintaining target blood sugar levels before conception is crucial to reduce the risk of complications.
- Medical Check-ups: Preconception consultations with healthcare providers to assess overall health and adjust medications if needed.

2. Continuous Blood Sugar Monitoring:

- Regular Monitoring: Increased frequency of blood sugar monitoring to track variations.
- Target Ranges: Tight glycemic control within specific target ranges to minimise risks.

3. Individualised Treatment Plans:

- Medication Adjustment: Modification of diabetes medications as needed, with a focus on safety for the developing foetus.
- Insulin Therapy: Insulin is often the preferred choice, and its dosage may be adjusted based on blood sugar levels.

4. Nutritional Management:

- Balanced Diet: Emphasis on a well-balanced diet to meet nutritional needs for both mother and baby.
- Carbohydrate Monitoring: Monitoring and controlling carbohydrate intake to manage blood sugar levels.

5. Regular Prenatal Check-ups:

- Medical Surveillance: Regular prenatal appointments to monitor both maternal and foetal health.
- Ultrasound Scans: Periodic ultrasound scans to assess the baby's growth and development.

6. Diabetes Education and Support:

- Educational Programs: Participation in diabetes education programs to enhance understanding of pregnancy-related diabetes management.
- Support Groups: Joining support groups or seeking psychological support to cope with the emotional aspects of managing diabetes during pregnancy.

7. Complication Prevention:

- Prevention of Gestational Diabetes: Monitoring and managing gestational diabetes if it develops during pregnancy.
- Blood Pressure Control: Managing blood pressure to prevent complications like preeclampsia.

8. Labour and Delivery Planning:

- Birth Plan: Collaborating with healthcare providers to create a birth plan that addresses specific diabetes-related considerations.
- Blood Sugar Monitoring during Labor: Continuous monitoring during labour to manage blood sugar levels.

9. Postpartum Care:

- Blood Sugar Monitoring After Birth: Continued monitoring of blood sugar levels after delivery.
- Breastfeeding: Guidance on managing diabetes while breastfeeding, including adjustments in insulin or medication as needed.

CHAPTER 3

Diagnosing Diabetes

Diagnosing diabetes involves a combination of clinical assessments and laboratory tests to determine blood sugar levels and assess the body's ability to regulate glucose. Early and accurate diagnosis is crucial for effective management. Here is an overview of the diagnostic process for diabetes:

1. Blood Sugar Tests:

- Fasting Blood Sugar (FBS):
    - Procedure: Blood sample taken after an overnight fast.
    - Diagnostic Criteria: Fasting blood sugar level of 126 milligrams per deciliter (mg/dL) or higher on two separate occasions indicates diabetes.
- Oral Glucose Tolerance Test (OGTT):
    - Procedure: Fasting blood sugar measured, followed by consumption of a glucose solution, and blood sugar levels tested at intervals.
    - Diagnostic Criteria: Blood sugar level of 200 mg/dL or higher two hours after consuming the glucose solution confirms diabetes.
- Random Blood Sugar Test:
    - Procedure: Blood sample taken at any time, regardless of the last meal.
    - Diagnostic Criteria: A blood sugar level of 200 mg/dL or higher, along with symptoms of diabetes, suggests diabetes.

2. A1C Test:

- Procedure: Measures the average blood sugar levels over the past 2-3 months.
- Diagnostic Criteria: A1C level of 6.5% or higher indicates diabetes.

3. Interpreting Test Results:

- Normal Range: Fasting blood sugar levels below 100 mg/dL, A1C levels below 5.7%.
- Pre-diabetes Range: Fasting blood sugar levels between 100-125 mg/dL, A1C levels between 5.7-6.4%.
- Diabetes Range: Fasting blood sugar levels of 126 mg/dL or higher, A1C levels of 6.5% or higher.

4. Confirmatory Testing:

- Repeat Tests: In cases where initial results are borderline, repeat testing may be recommended for confirmation.
- Different Tests: Utilising different types of blood sugar tests to cross-verify results.

5. Targeted Testing:

- Risk Factors: Testing may be recommended for individuals with risk factors such as family history, obesity, or a history of gestational diabetes.
- Symptoms: Diagnostic testing is warranted if individuals exhibit symptoms like excessive thirst, frequent urination, unexplained weight loss, or fatigue.

6. Monitoring during Pregnancy:

- Gestational Diabetes Testing: Pregnant women typically undergo glucose screening tests, like the glucose challenge test and OGTT, to assess gestational diabetes risk.

7. Diagnostic Guidelines:

- American Diabetes Association (ADA): ADA provides guidelines for the diagnosis of diabetes, emphasising the use of multiple tests for confirmation.

CHAPTER 4

Living with Diabetes

Living with diabetes requires a holistic approach that encompasses self-care, lifestyle adjustments, and ongoing management to maintain optimal health. Here's an overview of key aspects involved in living with diabetes:

1. Daily Blood Sugar Monitoring:

- Importance: Regular monitoring helps individuals understand how food, physical activity, and medication impact blood sugar levels.

- Devices: Utilising glucose metres and continuous glucose monitoring (CGM) systems for real-time feedback.

2. Medications and Insulin:

- Adherence: Following prescribed medication regimens and insulin schedules as directed by healthcare professionals.
- Adjustments: Collaborating with healthcare providers to adjust medications based on changing needs.

3. Meal Planning:

- Balanced Diet: Embracing a well-balanced diet rich in whole foods, fibre, and low in processed sugars and saturated fats.
- Carbohydrate Counting: Managing portion sizes and carbohydrate intake for better blood sugar control.

4. Exercise and Physical Activity:

- Benefits: Engaging in regular physical activity helps improve insulin sensitivity, manage weight, and enhance overall well-being.
- Customization: Tailoring exercise routines to individual preferences and physical abilities.

5. Stress Management:

- Impact on Blood Sugar: Recognizing the influence of stress on blood sugar levels and implementing stress-reduction techniques.
- Mindfulness: Incorporating mindfulness, meditation, or relaxation exercises into daily routines.

6. Regular Healthcare Check-ups:

- Routine Visits: Regular visits to healthcare professionals for diabetes management reviews.
- Screening for Complications: Periodic screening for diabetes-related complications, including eye exams, kidney function tests, and foot examinations.

7. Diabetes Education:

- Lifelong Learning: Continuous learning about diabetes management, new treatment options, and advancements in technology.
- Self-Empowerment: Gaining knowledge to make informed decisions about lifestyle, medications, and overall health.

8. Support Systems:

- Family and Friends: Building a strong support network with family and friends who understand and encourage diabetes management.
- Support Groups: Participating in diabetes support groups to connect with others facing similar challenges.

9. Emotional and Psychological Well-being:

- Coping Strategies: Developing effective coping mechanisms for the emotional impact of living with a chronic condition.
- Professional Support: Seeking counselling or therapy when needed to address emotional well-being.

10. Emergency Preparedness:

- Emergency Plan: Having a plan in place for managing diabetes during emergencies or unforeseen circumstances.
- Medical ID: Wearing a medical ID bracelet or carrying a card to communicate diabetes status in case of emergencies.

Choosing a Glucose Metre: A Practical Guide

Introduction:

Selecting the right glucose metre is crucial for effective diabetes management. With various options available, consider the following factors to make an informed decision:

1. Accuracy:

- Key Consideration: Choose a metre with proven accuracy.
- Verification: Look for metres that meet industry standards and have undergone rigorous testing.

2. Ease of Use:

- User-Friendly Design: Opt for a metre with a straightforward interface and easy navigation.
- Large Display: A clear and easy-to-read display is beneficial, especially for those with visual impairments.

3. Size and Portability:

- Compact Design: Consider the portability of the metre, especially if you're frequently on the go.
- Ease of Carrying: Some metres come with convenient carrying cases or features for easy transportation.

4. Testing Speed:

- Rapid Results: Choose a metre that provides quick and efficient results.
- Testing Time: Consider the time required for the metre to deliver accurate readings.

5. Sample Size and Application:

- Small Blood Sample: Metres with smaller sample requirements are more comfortable for users.
- Alternate Site Testing: Some metres allow testing on alternative sites, such as the forearm or palm.

6. Connectivity and Data Management:

- Bluetooth Capability: Select metres that offer Bluetooth connectivity for seamless data transfer to smartphones or other devices.
- Data Storage: Look for metres with sufficient memory to store a history of blood sugar readings.

7. Cost and Insurance Coverage:

- Affordability: Consider the overall cost of the metre, including test strips and accessories.
- Insurance Coverage: Check with your insurance provider for coverage options for specific metre models.

8. Test Strip Cost:

- Affordability of Strips: The ongoing cost of test strips can significantly impact your budget.
- Availability: Ensure that test strips are readily available and accessible.

9. Additional Features:

- Backlit Display: Useful for testing in low-light conditions.
- Reminder Alarms: Metres with reminder features can be beneficial for timely testing.

10. Customer Support and Resources:

- Manufacturer Support: Consider the reputation and customer support provided by the metre manufacturer.
- Educational Resources: Look for metres that offer educational materials and resources for users.

11. Integration with Other Devices:

- Compatibility: Choose a metre that can integrate with other diabetes management devices, such as insulin pumps or continuous glucose monitoring systems.

12. User Reviews:

- User Feedback: Read reviews from other users to understand their experiences with the metre.
- Reputation: Consider metres with positive reviews and a good reputation in the diabetes community.

Target Blood Sugar Ranges for Diabetes Management:

Maintaining blood sugar levels within specific target ranges is crucial for effective diabetes management. Individual targets may vary based on factors such as age, overall health, and the presence of other medical conditions. It's important to work closely with healthcare professionals to establish personalised goals. Here are general guidelines for target blood sugar ranges:

1. Fasting Blood Sugar (FBS):

- Normal Range: Below 100 mg/dL.
- Pre-diabetes Range: 100-125 mg/dL.
- Diabetes Range: 126 mg/dL or higher.

2. Postprandial Blood Sugar (2 hours after a meal):

- Normal Range: Below 140 mg/dL.
- Pre-diabetes Range: 140-199 mg/dL.
- Diabetes Range: 200 mg/dL or higher.

3. A1C (Haemoglobin A1C):

- Normal Range: Below 5.7%.
- Pre-diabetes Range: 5.7-6.4%.

- Diabetes Range: 6.5% or higher.

4. Before Meals (Preprandial):

- Target Range: 80-130 mg/dL.

5. Bedtime (Nighttime):

- Target Range: 90-150 mg/dL.

6. Target for Pregnant Individuals (Gestational Diabetes):

- Fasting: Below 95 mg/dL.
- 1 hour after meals: Below 140 mg/dL.

Important Considerations:

1. Individualization:

- Blood sugar targets should be personalised based on individual health factors, age, and specific medical conditions.

2. Variability:

- Recognize that blood sugar levels naturally fluctuate throughout the day, influenced by meals, physical activity, stress, and other factors.

3. Adjustments for Children:

- Paediatric blood sugar targets may differ, and adjustments should be made in consultation with paediatric healthcare providers.

4. Clinical Monitoring:

- Regular monitoring of blood sugar levels, along with discussions with healthcare providers, is crucial to assess and adjust targets as needed.

5. Risk of Hypoglycemia:

- Lowering blood sugar levels too aggressively may increase the risk of hypoglycemia (low blood sugar). Individualised goals should consider the balance between glucose control and avoiding hypoglycemic events.

6. Target Adjustments for Older Adults:

- Targets may be adjusted for older adults, considering factors such as cognitive function, overall health, and the risk of hypoglycemia.

Medications and Insulin in Diabetes Management:

Managing diabetes often involves a combination of medications, insulin therapy, and lifestyle modifications. The choice of treatment depends on the type of diabetes, individual health factors, and the effectiveness of each approach. Here's an overview of common medications and insulin used in diabetes management:

1. Type 1 Diabetes:

- Insulin Therapy:
    - Basal Insulin: Provides a steady release of insulin to control blood sugar levels between meals and during periods of fasting.
    - Bolus Insulin: Administered before meals to manage the increase in blood sugar after eating.

2. Type 2 Diabetes:

- Oral Medications:
    - Metformin: Improves insulin sensitivity and reduces glucose production by the liver.
    - Sulfonylureas: Stimulate the pancreas to release more insulin.
    - DPP-4 Inhibitors: Increase insulin release and decrease glucose production.

- GLP-1 Receptor Agonists: Stimulate insulin release, reduce glucagon production, and slow stomach emptying.
  - SGLT-2 Inhibitors: Block glucose reabsorption in the kidneys, leading to increased glucose excretion.
- Injectable Medications:
  - Insulin: Used in some cases when oral medications are insufficient to control blood sugar levels.
  - GLP-1 Receptor Agonists (Injectable): Mimic the action of GLP-1, promoting insulin release and reducing glucagon production.

3. Gestational Diabetes:

- Insulin: Often recommended for managing blood sugar levels during pregnancy.

4. Other Medications:

- Alpha-glucosidase Inhibitors: Slow the absorption of carbohydrates from the digestive tract.
- Meglitinides: Stimulate insulin release from the pancreas.
- Bile Acid Sequestrants: Used to lower blood sugar levels.

Important Considerations:

1. Individualised Treatment:

- Treatment plans are personalised based on factors such as age, overall health, lifestyle, and the presence of other medical conditions.

2. Insulin Types:

- Different types of insulin are available, including rapid-acting, short-acting, intermediate-acting, and long-acting. The choice depends on individual needs and preferences.

3. Combination Therapy:

- Some individuals may require a combination of medications to achieve optimal blood sugar control.

4. Monitoring and Adjustments:

- Regular monitoring of blood sugar levels is crucial for assessing the effectiveness of medications and making adjustments as needed.

5. Side Effects:

- Medications may have side effects, and healthcare providers monitor for potential issues while ensuring benefits outweigh risks.

6. Lifestyle Modifications:

- Medications work best when combined with a healthy diet, regular exercise, and other lifestyle modifications.

7. Insulin Delivery Devices:

- Insulin can be administered via insulin pens, syringes, or insulin pumps, providing flexibility in dosing.

8. Continuous Glucose Monitoring (CGM):

- CGM systems offer real-time data on blood sugar levels, assisting in the fine-tuning of medication and insulin regimens.

Creating a Diabetes Management Plan: A Comprehensive Guide

Managing diabetes effectively involves creating a personalised plan that addresses various aspects of daily life. A well-rounded diabetes management plan encompasses lifestyle modifications, medication adherence, monitoring, and regular communication with healthcare professionals. Here's a comprehensive guide to help create a diabetes management plan:

1. Collaborate with Healthcare Professionals:

- Medical Team: Establish a strong partnership with healthcare providers, including endocrinologists, primary care physicians, dietitians, and diabetes educators.
- Regular Check-ups: Schedule regular check-ups to assess overall health, adjust treatment plans, and address any concerns.

2. Understand Your Diabetes:

- Type of Diabetes: Clearly understand whether you have type 1, type 2, gestational diabetes, or another form, as management strategies may differ.
- Individual Factors: Consider personal health history, lifestyle, and any concurrent medical conditions.

3. Set Blood Sugar Targets:

- Consultation: Work with healthcare providers to establish personalised target ranges for fasting, postprandial, and A1C levels.
- Adjustments: Periodically reassess and adjust targets based on individual health goals and needs.

4. Develop a Healthy Eating Plan:

- Balanced Diet: Embrace a balanced diet rich in whole foods, fibre, fruits, vegetables, lean proteins, and whole grains.

- Portion Control: Monitor portion sizes and consider carbohydrate counting to manage blood sugar levels.

5. Regular Physical Activity:

- Exercise Routine: Develop an exercise routine that includes aerobic activities, strength training, and flexibility exercises.
- Consistency: Aim for regular physical activity to improve insulin sensitivity and overall well-being.

6. Medication Adherence:

- Understand Medications: Know the purpose, dosage, and potential side effects of medications prescribed.
- Adherence: Consistently take medications as prescribed, and communicate with healthcare providers about any concerns.

7. Blood Sugar Monitoring:

- Regular Testing: Establish a routine for blood sugar monitoring using a glucose metre or continuous glucose monitoring (CGM) system.
- Record Keeping: Keep a log of blood sugar levels, meals, and physical activity to identify patterns.

8. Develop a Sick Day Plan:

- Guidelines: Create a plan for managing diabetes during illness, including adjustments to medications, hydration, and monitoring.
- Communication: Know when to seek medical attention and inform healthcare providers about any illness.

9. Stress Management:

- Techniques: Incorporate stress-reduction techniques such as mindfulness, meditation, deep breathing, or hobbies into daily life.
- Counselling: Seek professional support if needed to address stress-related challenges.

10. Regular Eye, Foot, and Dental Exams:

- Screening: Schedule regular eye exams, foot checks, and dental appointments to detect and address diabetes-related complications early.

11. Emergency Preparedness:

- Emergency Kit: Create a diabetes emergency kit with essential supplies, medications, and contact information for healthcare providers.
- Education: Educate family members, friends, and colleagues about your diabetes management needs.

12. Join Support Groups:

- Community Connection: Consider joining diabetes support groups or online communities to share experiences, tips, and receive support.

13. Stay Informed:

- Ongoing Learning: Stay informed about advancements in diabetes management, new technologies, and treatment options.
- Continued Education: Participate in diabetes education programs for ongoing learning.

14. Regularly Review and Adjust:

- Periodic Assessment: Periodically review your diabetes management plan with healthcare providers to make adjustments based on changing needs.

- Lifestyle Changes: Adapt your plan to accommodate lifestyle changes, such as changes in physical activity, work, or living situations.

CHAPTER 5

Complications of Diabetes

Diabetes, if not effectively managed, can lead to various complications affecting different parts of the body. Proper blood sugar control, lifestyle modifications, and regular medical check-ups are crucial in preventing or managing these complications. Here's an overview of common complications associated with diabetes:

1. Cardiovascular Complications:

- Heart Disease: Individuals with diabetes have an increased risk of developing heart disease, including coronary artery disease, heart attacks, and heart failure.
- Stroke: Diabetes raises the risk of stroke due to the impact on blood vessels.

2. Eye Complications:

- Diabetic Retinopathy: Damage to blood vessels in the retina, leading to vision problems and potential blindness if left untreated.
- Cataracts and Glaucoma: Diabetes increases the risk of developing cataracts and glaucoma.

3. Neuropathy (Nerve Damage):

- Peripheral Neuropathy: Nerve damage affecting the extremities, leading to pain, tingling, numbness, and loss of sensation.
- Autonomic Neuropathy: Affects internal organs, leading to digestive, urinary, and cardiovascular issues.

4. Kidney Complications:

- Diabetic Nephropathy: Damage to the kidneys, potentially leading to kidney failure.
- Increased Blood Pressure: Diabetes can contribute to elevated blood pressure, further impacting kidney function.

5. Foot Complications:

- Peripheral Arterial Disease (PAD): Reduced blood flow to the lower extremities, increasing the risk of infections and slow wound healing.
- Foot Ulcers: Open sores or wounds on the feet that can lead to infections and, in severe cases, amputation.

6. Skin Complications:

- Bacterial and Fungal Infections: Diabetes can increase the risk of skin infections, especially if blood sugar levels are poorly controlled.
- Dry Skin and Itching: Diabetes may lead to dry skin, which is prone to itching and potential infection.

7. Dental and Gum Issues:

- Gingivitis and Periodontitis: Diabetes is associated with an increased risk of gum disease, which can affect oral health.
- Tooth Loss: Poorly controlled diabetes may contribute to tooth loss.

8. Sexual and Reproductive Complications:

- Erectile Dysfunction: Men with diabetes may experience difficulties with sexual function.
- Irregular Menstrual Cycles: Women with diabetes may face hormonal imbalances affecting menstrual cycles and fertility.

9. Mental Health Concerns:

- Depression and Anxiety: Diabetes management can be challenging, contributing to mental health issues.
- Cognitive Decline: Some studies suggest a link between diabetes and an increased risk of cognitive decline and dementia.

10. Increased Risk of Infections:

- Weakened Immune System: Diabetes can compromise the immune system, leading to an increased risk of infections, especially in the skin and urinary tract.

11. Increased Risk of Certain Cancers:

- Pancreatic Cancer: Individuals with diabetes may have an elevated risk of pancreatic cancer.
- Colorectal and Breast Cancer: Some studies suggest an association between diabetes and an increased risk of certain cancers.

Prevention and Management Strategies:

- Blood Sugar Control: Maintaining optimal blood sugar levels is paramount in preventing complications.
- Regular Check-ups: Periodic medical examinations, eye exams, and screenings for kidney function are essential.

- Healthy Lifestyle: Adopting a balanced diet, regular exercise, and avoiding smoking contribute to overall health.

Diabetic Retinopathy: Understanding the Eye Complication of Diabetes

Diabetic retinopathy is a serious eye condition that can affect individuals with diabetes. It results from damage to the blood vessels of the retina, the light-sensitive tissue at the back of the eye. Proper diabetes management and regular eye exams are essential in preventing and managing diabetic retinopathy. Here's an overview of this eye complication:

1. Causes:

- Prolonged High Blood Sugar: Elevated blood sugar levels over an extended period can lead to damage of the small blood vessels nourishing the retina.
- Hypertension: High blood pressure is a contributing factor to the progression of diabetic retinopathy.

2. Stages of Diabetic Retinopathy:

- Non-Proliferative Diabetic Retinopathy (NPDR): The early stage, characterised by microaneurysms, small haemorrhages, and retinal swelling.
- Proliferative Diabetic Retinopathy (PDR): Advanced stage where new blood vessels grow on the retina, which can lead to bleeding and scar tissue formation.

3. Symptoms:

- Early Stages (NPDR):
    - Often asymptomatic.
    - Blurred or fluctuating vision.
    - Difficulty perceiving colours.
- Advanced Stages (PDR):
    - Severe vision loss.

  - Floaters or spots in the field of vision.
  - Complete vision loss in extreme cases.

4. Risk Factors:

- Duration of Diabetes: The longer an individual has diabetes, the higher the risk.
- Poor Blood Sugar Control: Uncontrolled blood sugar levels contribute to retinopathy progression.
- Hypertension: High blood pressure increases the risk of complications.
- Genetics: Family history of diabetic retinopathy may elevate the risk.

5. Prevention and Management:

- Regular Eye Exams: Annual comprehensive eye exams are crucial for early detection and intervention.
- Blood Sugar Control: Maintaining optimal blood sugar levels helps prevent and slow the progression of retinopathy.
- Blood Pressure Management: Controlling hypertension is essential in reducing the risk of complications.
- Lifestyle Modifications: Adopting a healthy lifestyle, including a balanced diet and regular exercise, contributes to overall eye health.

6. Treatment Options:

- Laser Photocoagulation: Laser therapy to seal or shrink abnormal blood vessels and reduce swelling.
- Anti-VEGF Injections: Medications injected into the eye to inhibit the growth of abnormal blood vessels.
- Vitrectomy: Surgical removal of blood from the vitreous gel in the eye in advanced cases.

7. Importance of Early Intervention:

- Early Detection: Regular eye exams allow for the early detection of diabetic retinopathy.
- Timely Treatment: Prompt treatment in the early stages can prevent or slow progression.

8. Living with Diabetic Retinopathy:

- Adaptations: Individuals with advanced stages may need to adapt to visual changes.
- Support Systems: Emotional and practical support from family and healthcare professionals is crucial.

CHAPTER 6

Special Considerations

Special Considerations in Diabetes Management: Addressing Unique Needs

Managing diabetes involves considering individualised factors that may impact treatment and care. Certain populations, such as older adults, children, pregnant individuals, and those with comorbidities, require special considerations. Here's an overview of key considerations for these groups:

1. Older Adults:

- Cognitive Function: Consider cognitive function when developing treatment plans, ensuring that older adults can manage medications and monitor blood sugar effectively.
- Polypharmacy: Be mindful of potential interactions with other medications, as older adults may be taking multiple drugs for various health conditions.
- Frailty and Mobility: Assess physical limitations and adapt diabetes management strategies accordingly, especially in terms of exercise and lifestyle modifications.

2. Children and Adolescents:

- Growth and Development: Adjust insulin regimens and treatment plans to accommodate growth spurts and changes in physical activity levels.
- Family Involvement: Engage families in diabetes management, providing education and support to ensure proper care for children.
- Psychosocial Aspects: Address the emotional and social impact of diabetes on children and adolescents, promoting a positive attitude toward self-care.

3. Pregnant Individuals with Diabetes:

- Preconception Planning: Encourage preconception planning to optimise blood sugar levels before pregnancy.
- Gestational Diabetes: Monitor and manage gestational diabetes to reduce the risk of complications for both the mother and the baby.
- Collaborative Care: Coordinate care among obstetricians, endocrinologists, and diabetes educators to ensure comprehensive support.

4. Individuals with Comorbidities:

- Cardiovascular Disease: Manage diabetes in conjunction with cardiovascular risk factors, focusing on blood pressure and cholesterol control.
- Kidney Disease: Adjust medications and treatment plans to account for compromised kidney function, monitoring closely for potential complications.
- Mental Health Conditions: Address the impact of diabetes on mental health, considering the bidirectional relationship between diabetes and conditions such as depression.

5. Cultural and Socioeconomic Considerations:

- Dietary Preferences: Recognize and respect cultural dietary preferences while providing guidance on healthy eating.
- Access to Healthcare: Consider socioeconomic factors that may impact access to medications, healthcare services, and diabetes education.

6. Technological Considerations:

- Technology Adoption: Assess the willingness and ability of individuals to use technological tools, such as continuous glucose monitoring (CGM) systems or insulin pumps.
- Digital Literacy: Provide education and support for individuals to navigate and benefit from digital health resources.

7. Individualised Education and Support:

- Tailored Education: Customise diabetes education to meet the unique needs of each individual, considering factors such as health literacy and cultural background.
- Peer Support: Foster connections with peer support groups, allowing individuals to share experiences and learn from others facing similar challenges.

8. Transitions in Care:

- Paediatric to Adult Care: Facilitate a smooth transition from paediatric to adult diabetes care, addressing the evolving needs and responsibilities of the individual.
- Hospital Discharges: Ensure clear communication and coordination between healthcare providers during hospitalizations to maintain continuity of care.

CHAPTER 7

Emotional and Psychological Aspects

Living with diabetes involves not only managing physical health but also addressing the emotional and psychological aspects of the condition. The impact of diabetes on mental well-being is significant, and a holistic approach to care should encompass emotional support, coping strategies, and mental health awareness. Here's an overview of the emotional and psychological aspects of diabetes:

1. Emotional Impact:

- Diagnosis Reaction: Individuals may experience a range of emotions, including shock, fear, sadness, or even relief upon receiving a diabetes diagnosis.
- Stigma and Misconceptions: Addressing societal stigma and dispelling misconceptions about diabetes can help alleviate emotional distress.

2. Stress Management:

- Influence on Blood Sugar: Stress can affect blood sugar levels, emphasising the need for effective stress management techniques.
- Mindfulness and Relaxation: Encourage practices such as mindfulness, deep breathing, and relaxation exercises to reduce stress.

3. Anxiety and Depression:

- Prevalence: Individuals with diabetes may be at a higher risk of anxiety and depression.
- Screening: Regular screening for mental health conditions is essential, with timely intervention and support.

4. Coping Strategies:

- Problem-solving: Develop effective problem-solving skills to address challenges related to diabetes management.
- Positive Coping: Encourage positive coping mechanisms, such as seeking support, maintaining a healthy lifestyle, and engaging in activities that bring joy.

5. Diabetes Burnout:

- Definition: Diabetes burnout refers to the emotional and physical exhaustion that can result from the constant demands of managing the condition.
- Recognizing Signs: Be aware of signs of burnout, such as neglecting self-care or feeling overwhelmed, and provide support and resources.

6. Support Systems:

- Family and Friends: Involving family and friends in diabetes care can create a strong support network.
- Support Groups: Joining diabetes support groups provides opportunities to connect with others facing similar challenges and share experiences.

7. Communication:

- Open Dialogue: Encourage open communication between individuals with diabetes and their healthcare providers to address emotional concerns.
- Family Communication: Facilitate communication within families to promote understanding and support.

8. Goal Setting and Motivation:

- Setting Realistic Goals: Help individuals set achievable and realistic goals for diabetes management.
- Celebrating Achievements: Acknowledge and celebrate successes, no matter how small, to boost motivation.

9. Educating Loved Ones:

- Family Education: Educate family members about diabetes, fostering empathy and understanding.
- School and Workplace Awareness: Raise awareness in school and workplace settings to create supportive environments.

10. Professional Mental Health Support:

- Counselling and Therapy: Consider incorporating counselling or therapy for individuals struggling with emotional and psychological challenges.
- Collaboration with Mental Health Professionals: Collaborate with mental health professionals to provide comprehensive care.

11. Continuous Learning:

- Diabetes Education Programs: Encourage participation in diabetes education programs to enhance knowledge and skills.
- Staying Informed: Regularly update individuals on advancements in diabetes management and mental health resources.

CHAPTER 8

Advances in Diabetes Research and Technology

Recent years have witnessed remarkable strides in diabetes research and technology, revolutionising the landscape of diabetes management. These advancements aim to improve treatment outcomes, enhance patient experience, and empower individuals living with diabetes. Here are key areas of progress in diabetes research and technology:

1. Continuous Glucose Monitoring (CGM):

- Real-Time Data: CGM systems provide real-time information about glucose levels, helping individuals make immediate and informed decisions about insulin dosing and lifestyle.
- Alerts and Trends: Advanced CGM devices offer customizable alerts for high and low glucose levels, as well as insights into glucose trends over time.

2. Artificial Pancreas Systems:

- Closed-Loop Systems: Combining CGM with insulin pumps, artificial pancreas systems automatically adjust insulin delivery in response to real-time glucose readings.
- Improved Stability: These systems aim to maintain more stable blood sugar levels, reducing the risk of hypoglycemia and hyperglycemia.

3. Insulin Delivery Devices:

- Smart Insulin Pens: Digital insulin pens offer features such as dose tracking, Bluetooth connectivity, and data synchronisation with mobile apps.
- Patch Insulin Delivery: Wearable patch pumps provide discreet and continuous insulin delivery, eliminating the need for injections.

4. Advanced Insulin Formulations:

- Ultra-Rapid Insulin: Formulations with quicker onset and shorter duration, mimicking the body's natural insulin response.
- Long-Acting Insulin Analogs: Extended-release formulations with prolonged action, reducing the frequency of injections.

5. Telemedicine and Remote Monitoring:

- Virtual Consultations: Telemedicine facilitates remote consultations with healthcare providers, improving accessibility to diabetes care.
- Remote Monitoring Devices: Devices that allow healthcare providers to remotely access and monitor patients' glucose data for timely interventions.

6. Precision Medicine:

- Genetic and Biomarker Research: Advances in understanding individual genetic and biomarker profiles contribute to personalised treatment approaches.
- Tailored Therapies: Precision medicine aims to tailor diabetes management strategies based on an individual's unique characteristics and response to treatment.

7. Smart Insulin and Glucose-Sensing Technologies:

- Responsive Insulin: Smart insulin formulations that adjust their activity in response to glucose levels, providing a more dynamic approach to blood sugar control.
- Implantable Sensors: Miniaturised, implantable sensors that continuously monitor glucose levels and communicate wirelessly with external devices.

8. Gene Therapy and Regenerative Medicine:

- Beta Cell Regeneration: Research explores ways to regenerate insulin-producing beta cells in the pancreas.
- Gene Editing Techniques: Advancements in gene therapy may offer new possibilities for modifying genes related to insulin regulation.

9. Digital Health Apps and Platforms:

- Diabetes Management Apps: Mobile applications offer features such as meal tracking, medication reminders, and glucose trend analysis.
- Integration with Wearables: Apps seamlessly integrate with wearable devices, enabling continuous health monitoring.

10. Advanced Data Analytics:

- Machine Learning and AI: Data analytics and artificial intelligence help process large datasets, offering insights into personalised treatment plans and predictive modelling for glucose trends.
- Decision Support Systems: Intelligent systems assist healthcare providers and individuals in making data-driven decisions for optimal diabetes management.

11. Automated Insulin Dosing Algorithms:

- Smart Algorithms: Automated algorithms help optimise insulin dosing based on individual data, contributing to precision in diabetes care.
- Improved Glycemic Control: These systems aim to achieve and maintain target glucose levels more effectively.

12. Prevention and Early Detection:

- Predictive Modelling: Research focuses on developing models that predict the risk of diabetes onset, allowing for preventive measures.
- Early Detection Tools: Technologies for early detection of diabetes-related complications, such as retinopathy and neuropathy.

I WISH YOU A QUICK RECOVERY. GOD BLESS YOU

www.ingramcontent.com/pod-product-compliance
Lightning Source LLC
Chambersburg PA
CBHW050750250726
48662CB00005B/2132